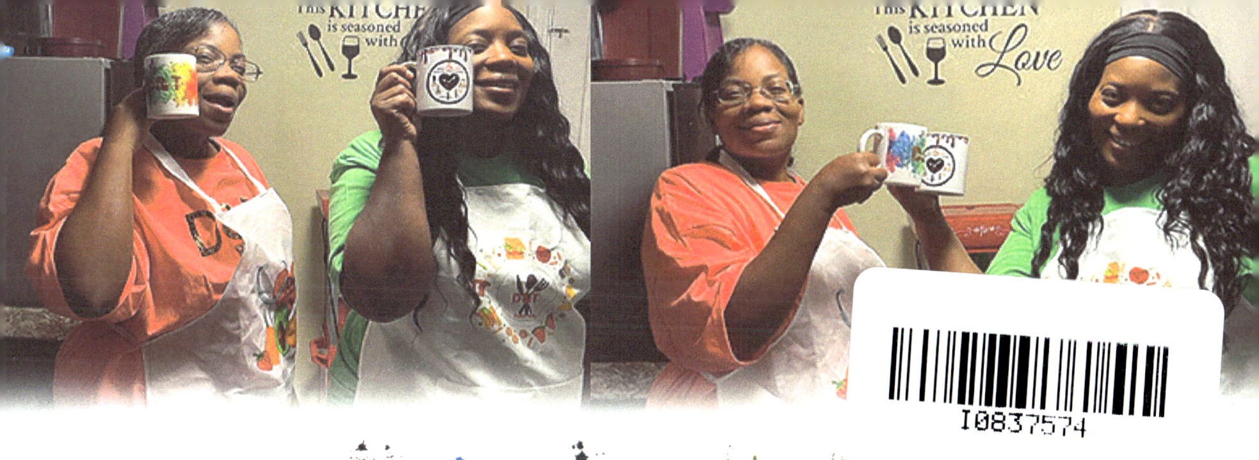

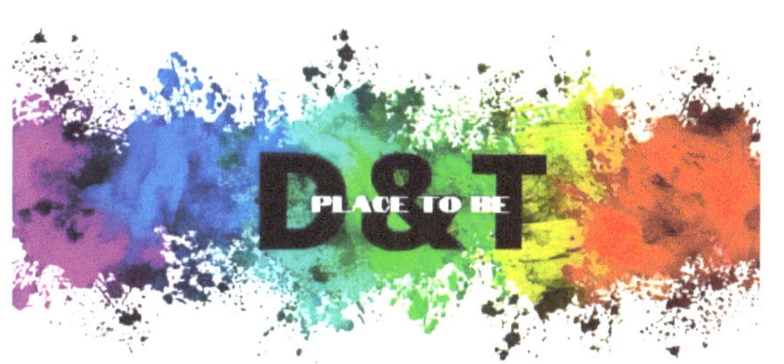

20 Delicious

Smoothie Recipes

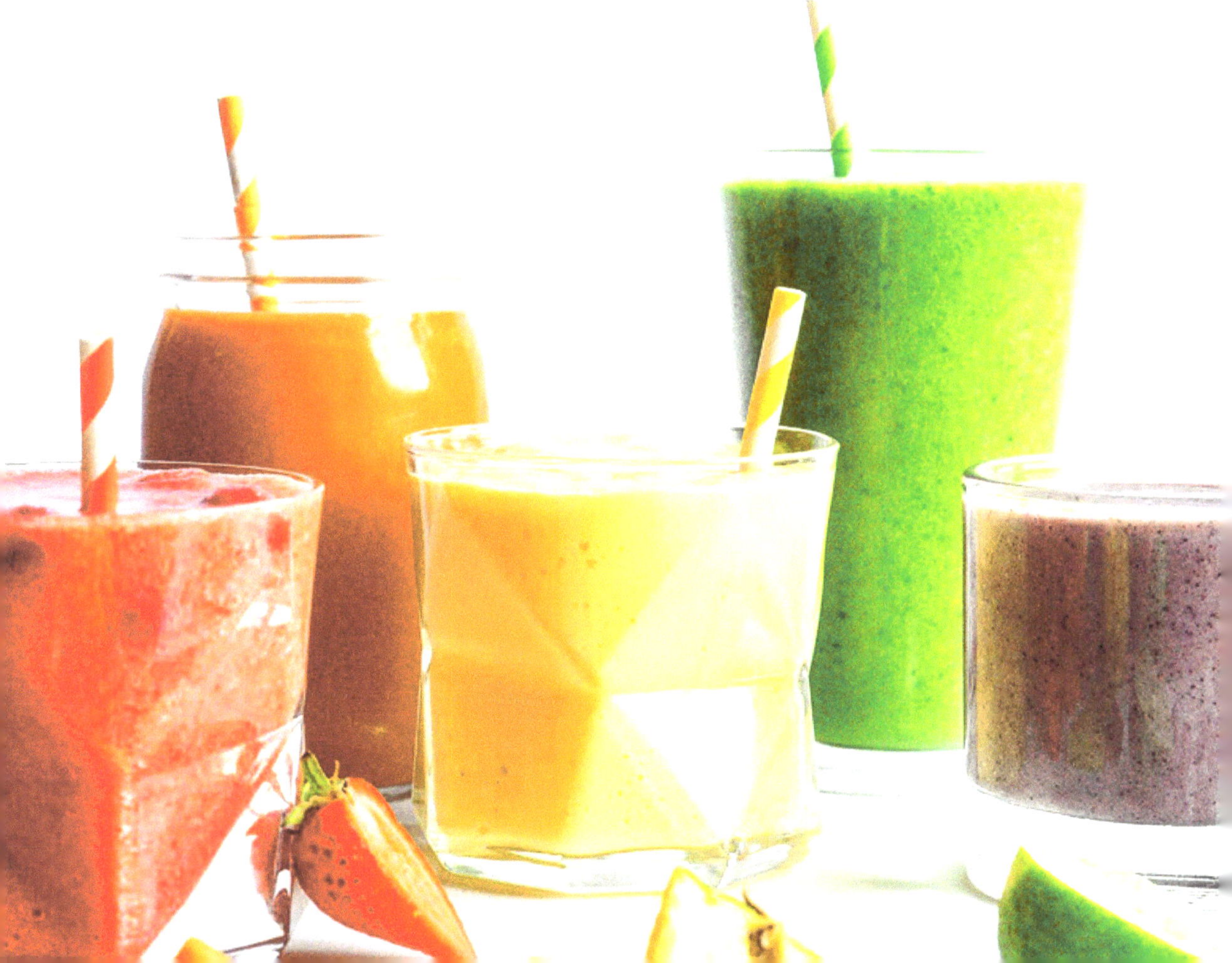

Table of Contents

NOURISHING SMOOTHIE RECIPE

Preparation time: 5 minutes
Serves: 2

This nutritious green smoothie recipe is specially created to increase the absorption of beneficial nutrients from various foods. It also provides probiotics, vitamins and minerals which are essential in proper food digestion and help in maintaining a healthy and functional digestive tract.

Ingredients:
1 cup vanilla almond milk
2 cups loosely packed kale
1 Granny Smith apple
1 avocado
1 organic lime, juiced
2 teaspoons raw honey

Directions: Mix together all ingredients in the blender. Pulse for 30 seconds on low speed, adjust to high and pulse until smooth. Serve immediately.

Nutrition Information (Per Serving):
Calorie: 288.5
Protein: 3.7g
Carbohydrate: 37g
Fat: 16.5g
Fiber: 10.5g
Sugar: 20g

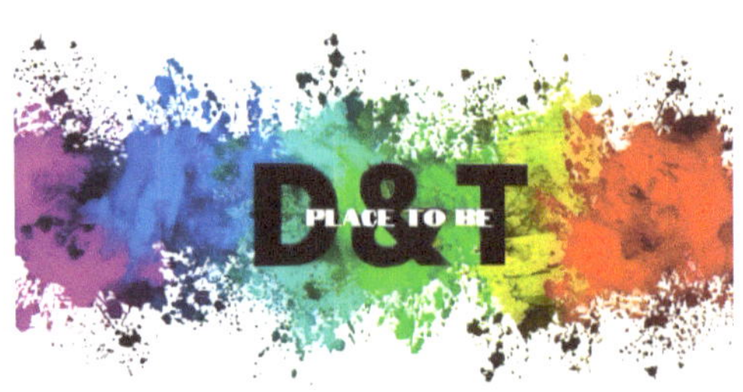

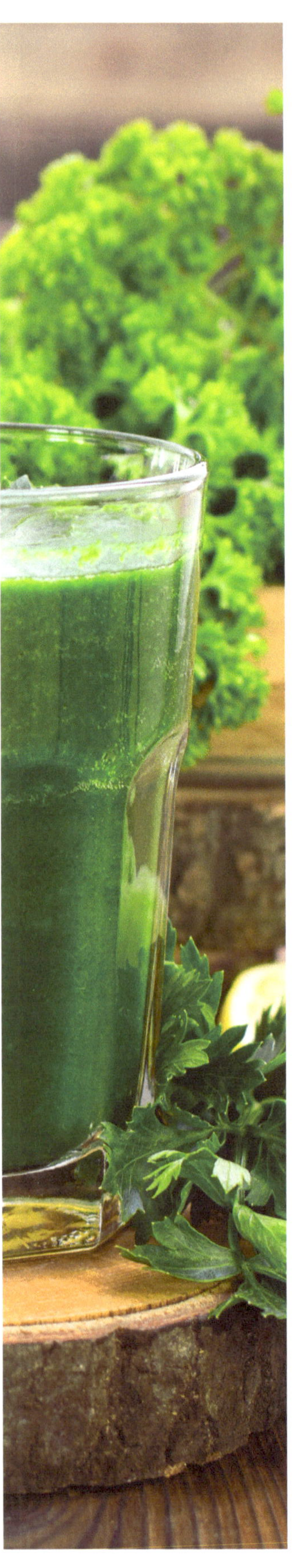

DETOX SMOOTHIE RECIPE

Preparation time: 5 minutes
Serves: 2

This detox smoothie recipe is rich fibre and antioxidants for body detox treatment. It is also aids in food digestion due to high amounts of fibre and maintains a healthy gut for effective nutrient absorption.

Ingredients:
½ cup orange juice
1 cup of coconut water (optional)
4 kernels of Brazil nuts
1 cup frozen pineapple chunks
1 cup loosely packed baby spinach
2 medium stalk of celery
1-inch piece lemongrass stalk
1 medium apple

Directions: Mix together all ingredients in the blender. Pulse for 30 seconds on low speed, adjust to high and pulse until smooth. Serve immediately.

Nutrition Information (Per Serving):
Calorie: 281
Protein: 4.2g
Carbohydrate: 58g
Fat: 7.5g
Fiber: 6g
Sugar: 34g

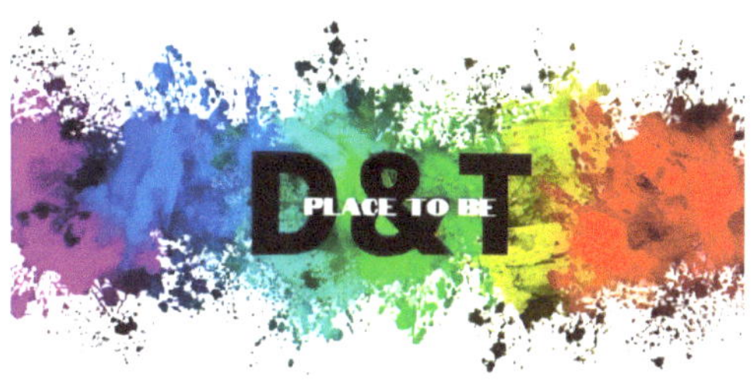

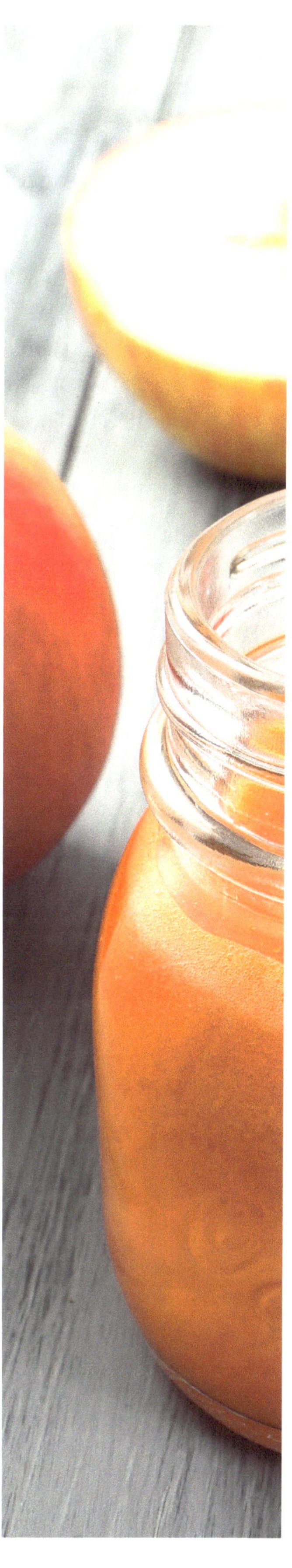

WEIGHT LOSS SMOOTHIE RECIPE

Preparation time: 5 minutes
Serves: 2

The ingredients used in this smoothie recipe are proven to help in loosing body weight and regulation. Due to its high satiety value, it helps decrease appetite and food cravings for effective body weight reduction.

Ingredients:
1 cup unsweetened almond milk
½ cup fresh pineapple juice
1 ripe banana
1 cup guava, seeded
1 cup diced frozen watermelon
2 cups packed baby spinach
1 tablespoon of raw honey

Directions: Mix together all ingredients in the blender. Pulse for 30 seconds on low speed, adjust to high and pulse until smooth. Serve immediately.

Nutrition Information (Per Serving):
Calorie: 185.5
Protein: 3.7g
Carbohydrate: 41.5g
Fat: 2.2g
Fiber: 4.1g
Sugar: 29.5g

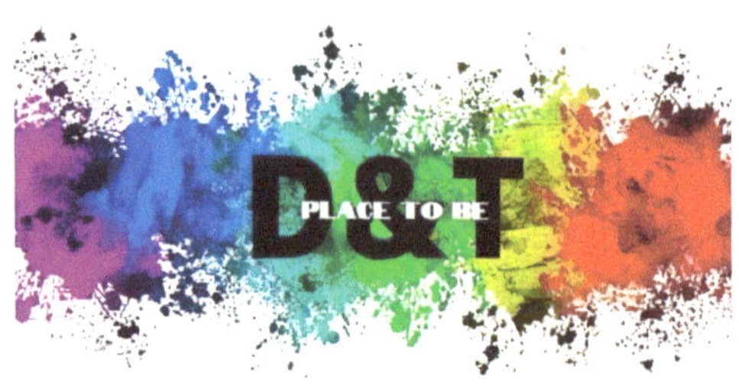

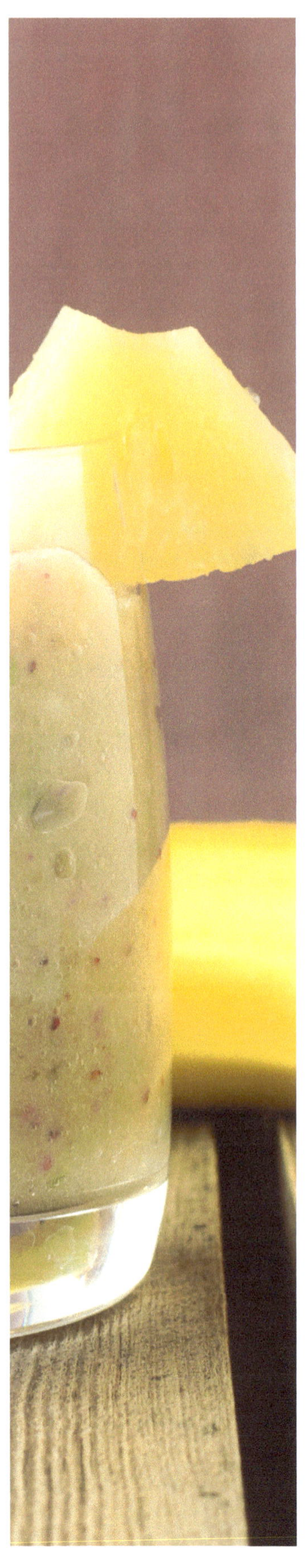

ANTI-AGING SMOOTHIE RECIPE

Preparation time: 5 minutes
Serves: 2

This delicious anti-aging smoothie recipe is packed with antioxidants and vitamins to keep a healthy and well-nourished skin. It provides Vitamin A, C and E with collagen and B-complex for firmer, younger and glowing skin.

Ingredients:
1 cup unsweetened almond milk
½ cup dairy free yogurt
2 kiwis
1 avocado
1 cup frozen blueberry
½ cup pomegranate arils
1 tablespoon maple syrup (optional

Directions: Mix together all ingredients in the blender. Pulse for 30 seconds on low speed, adjust to high and pulse until smooth. Serve immediately.

Nutrition Information (Per Serving):
Calorie: 298.5
Protein: 4.3g
Carbohydrate: 37.5g
Fat: 17g
Fiber: 13.5g
Sugar: 29g

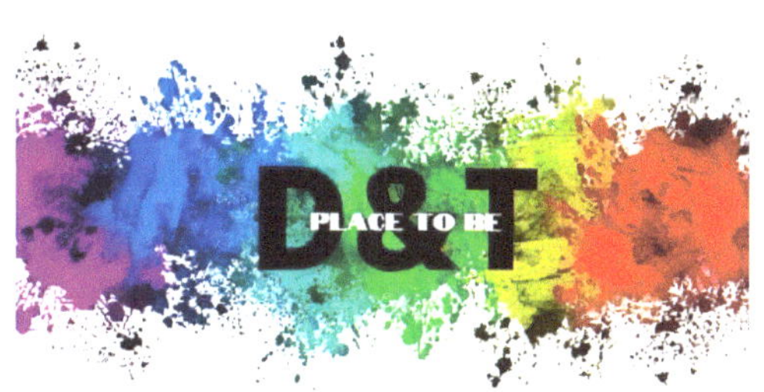

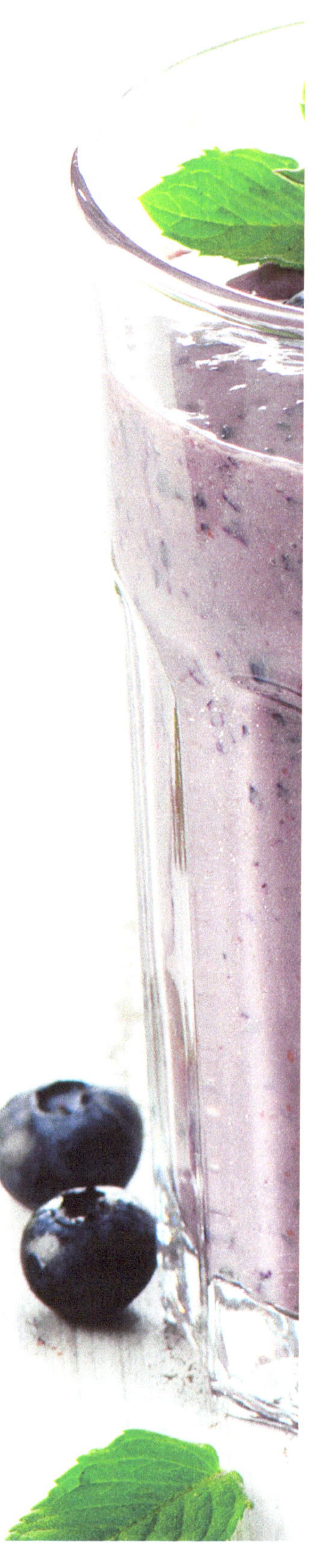

IMMUNE-BOOSTING SMOOTHIE

Preparation time: 5 minutes
Serves: 2

The ingredients in this Immune-boosting smoothie recipe provide beneficial nutrients for proper immune functioning, decreasing risk in cancer development and reducing excessive inflammatory reactions.

Ingredients:
½ cup cranberry juice
1 cup dairy free yogurt
1 orange, segmented
1 grapefruit, segmented
1 cup frozen blueberries
¼ cup dried Goji berries
2 cups loosely packed kale

Directions: Mix together all ingredients in the blender. Pulse for 30 seconds on low speed, adjust to high and pulse until smooth. Serve immediately.

Nutrition Information (Per Serving):
Calorie: 240
Protein: 15.5g
Carbohydrate: 45.5g
Fat: 1.1g
Fiber: 5.5g
Sugar: 25.5g

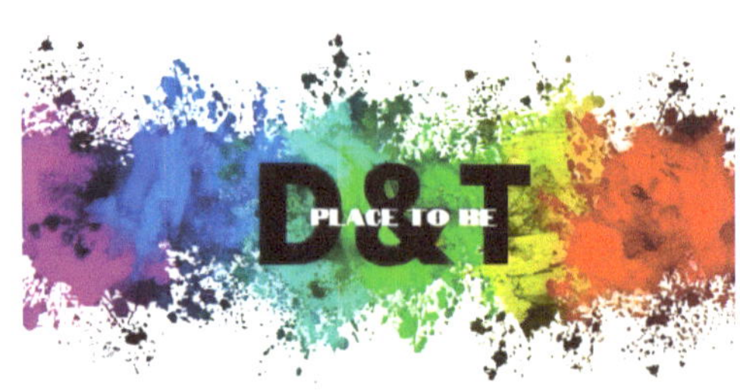

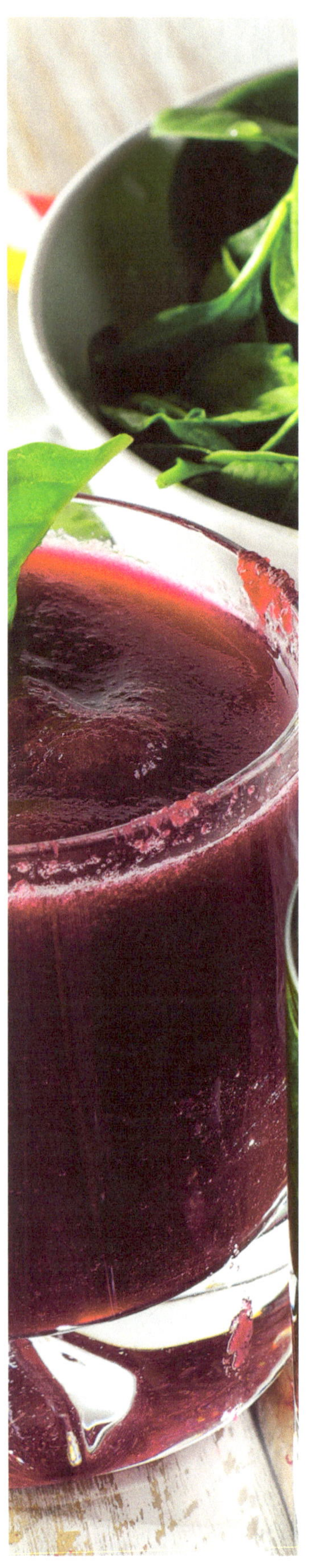

ENERGIZING SMOOTHIE RECIPE

Preparation time: 5 minutes
Serves: 2

This nutritious smoothie recipe is very filling and also helps in providing the body with high amounts of energy source.

Ingredients:
2 cups frozen raspberries
1 cup vanilla almond milk
2 tablespoons almond butter
1 ripe banana
2 cups loosely packed kale
1 orange, segmented
1 teaspoon raw honey

Directions: Mix together all ingredients in the blender. Pulse for 30 seconds on low speed, adjust to high and pulse until smooth. Serve immediately.

Nutrition Information (Per Serving):
Calorie: 276
Protein: 7.5g
Carbohydrate: 42g
Fat: 11.5g
Fiber: 13.5g
Sugar: 20g

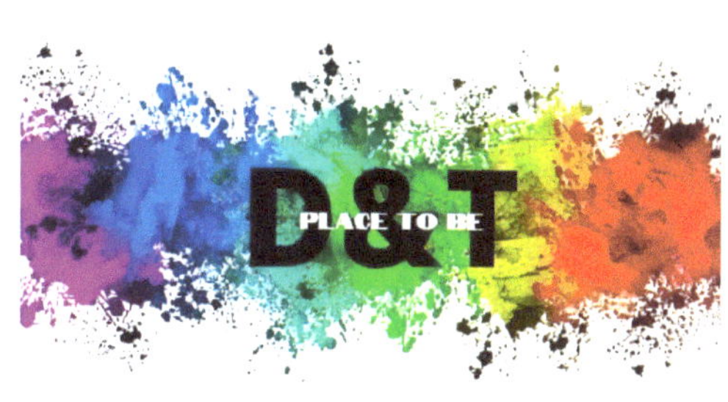

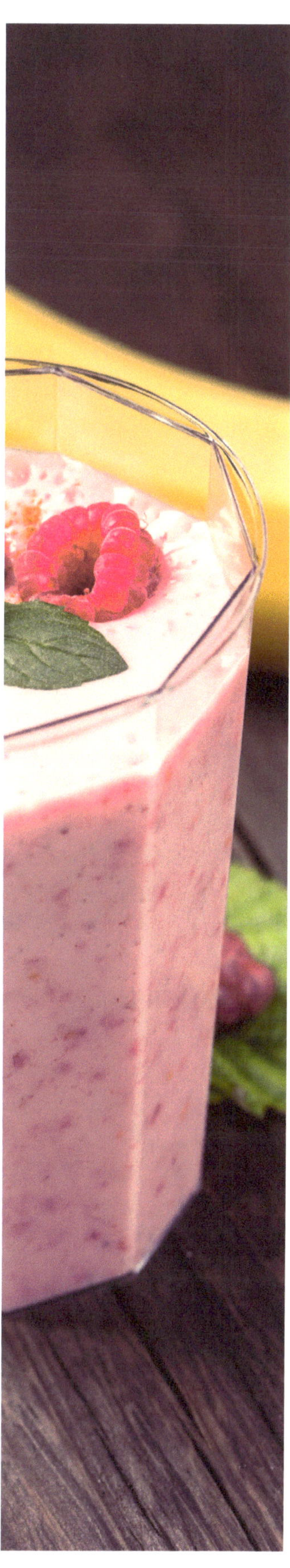

BRAIN-BOOSTING SMOOTHIE

Preparation time: 5 minutes
Serves: 2

With this special set of healthy and natural smoothie ingredients, it provides sufficient amounts of beneficial nutrients that help in improving memory, learning and all cognitive brain functions. This smoothie recipe keeps a healthy and functional brain and from free radical damage.

Ingredients:
4 almonds
1 cup coconut water
1 cup packed spinach
1 medium avocado
1 cup frozen blueberries
1 tablespoon chia seeds

Directions: Mix together all ingredients in the blender. Pulse for 30 seconds on low speed, adjust to high and pulse until smooth. Serve immediately.

Nutrition Information (Per Serving):
Calorie: 277.5
Protein: 5.5g
Carbohydrate: 30.5g
Fat: 33.5g
Fiber: 16g
Sugar: 9.5g

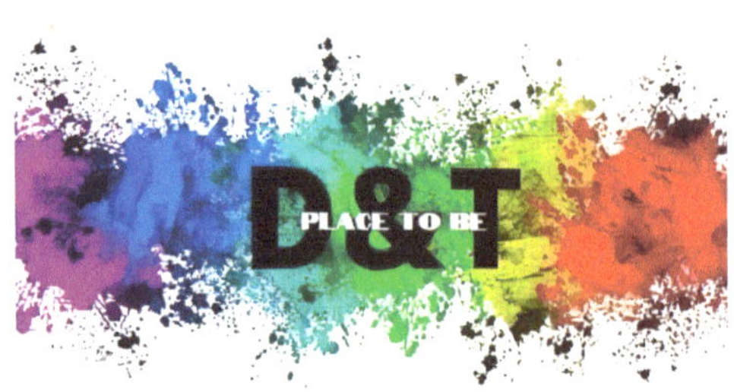

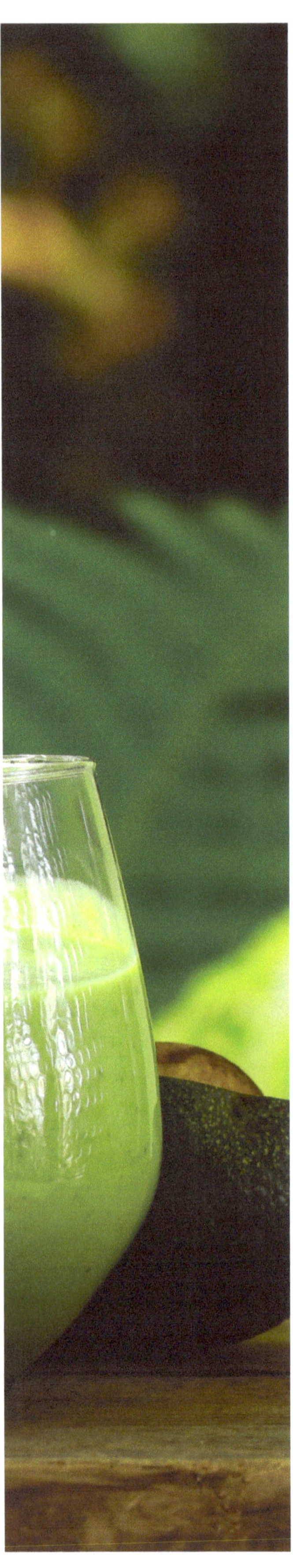

ANTI-INFLAMMATORY SMOOTHIE

Preparation time: 5 minutes
Serves: 2

This delicious smoothie recipe contains anti-inflammatory substances to help reduce and limit joint inflammations by blocking chemicals in the body that cause this auto-immune response.

Ingredients:
1 tablespoon hemp seeds
1 cup dairy free yogurt
½ cup cranberry juice (optional
2 cups frozen red raspberries
1 cup packed spinach
1-inch piece fresh ginger root
1 to 2 tablespoons of raw honey

Directions: Mix together all ingredients in the blender. Pulse for 30 seconds on low speed, adjust to high and pulse until smooth. Serve immediately.

Nutrition Information (Per Serving):
Calorie: 220.5
Protein: 15.5g
Carbohydrate: 36.5g
Fat: 3.8g
Fiber: 8.5g
Sugar: 25.5g

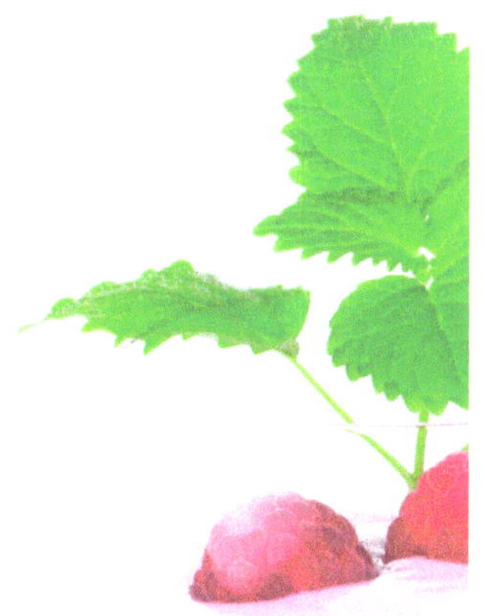

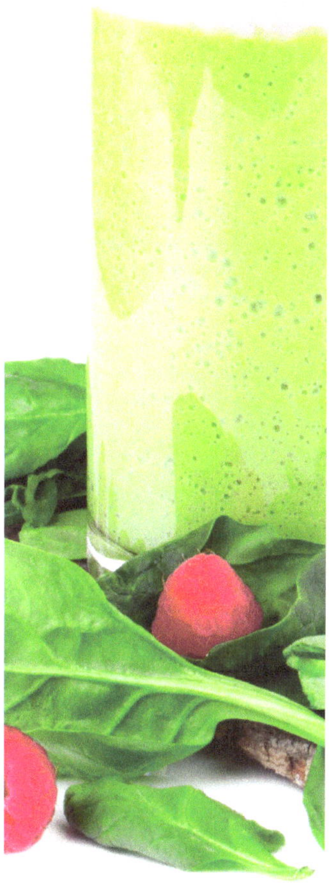

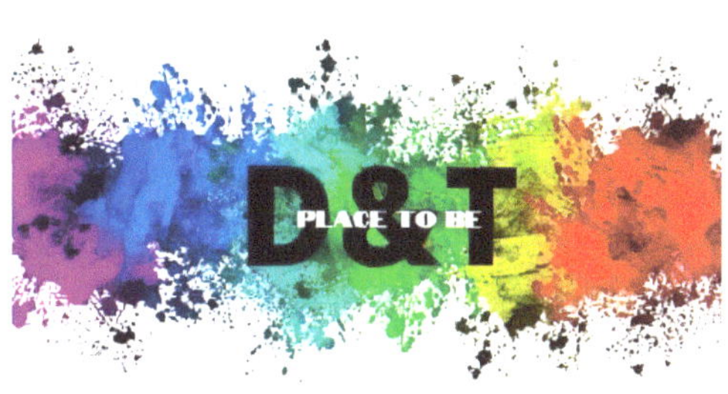

MUSCLE BUILDING SMOOTHIE

Preparation time: 5 minutes
Serves: 2

This nutritious green smoothie not only aids in building muscle but also helps in burning fats. It also helps restore spent energy and recover muscle injuries or damages from intensive physical activities.

Ingredients:
4 pitted prunes
1 tablespoon chia or hemp seeds
1 cup dairy free yogurt
2 cups loosely packed kale
2 fresh figs, trimmed
1 frozen ripe banana
1 pear

Directions: Mix together all ingredients in the blender. Pulse for 30 seconds on low speed, adjust to high and pulse until smooth. Serve immediately.

Nutrition Information (Per Serving):
Calorie: 286
Protein: 15g
Carbohydrate: 55g
Fat: 3.3g
Fiber: 9.5g
Sugar: 34g

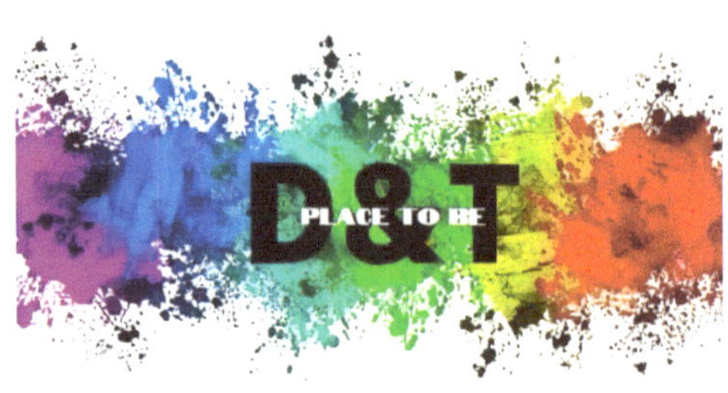

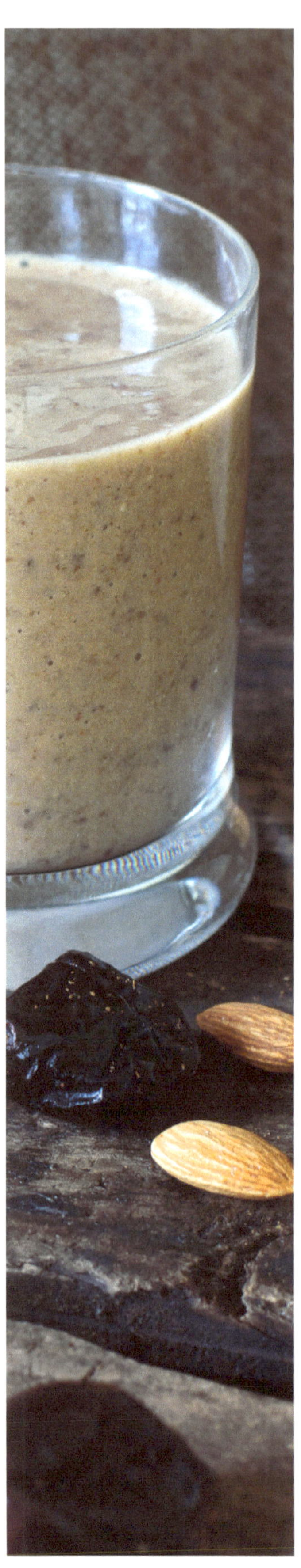

DIGESTIVE ENHANCER SMOOTHIE

Preparation time: 5 minutes
Serves: 2

This smoothie recipe promotes healthy digestion by stimulating the release of digestive enzymes for better gut functioning. When the gut is kept healthy and maintained in a functional state, it results to complete and effective food digestion necessary for improving nutritional health status of a person.

Ingredients:
1 kiwi
6 ounces dairy free yogurt
1 cup loosely packed kale
1 medium cucumber
1 medium avocado
1 tablespoon of organic lime juice
1 tablespoon of raw honey

Directions: Mix together all ingredients in the blender. Pulse for 30 seconds on low speed, adjust to high and pulse until smooth. Serve immediately.

Nutrition Information (Per Serving):
Calorie: 292.5
Protein: 22.5g
Carbohydrate: 32.5g
Fat: 15.5g
Fiber: 9g
Sugar: 18g

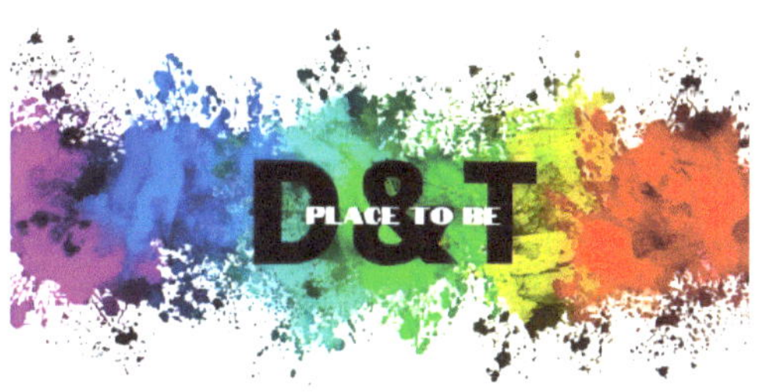

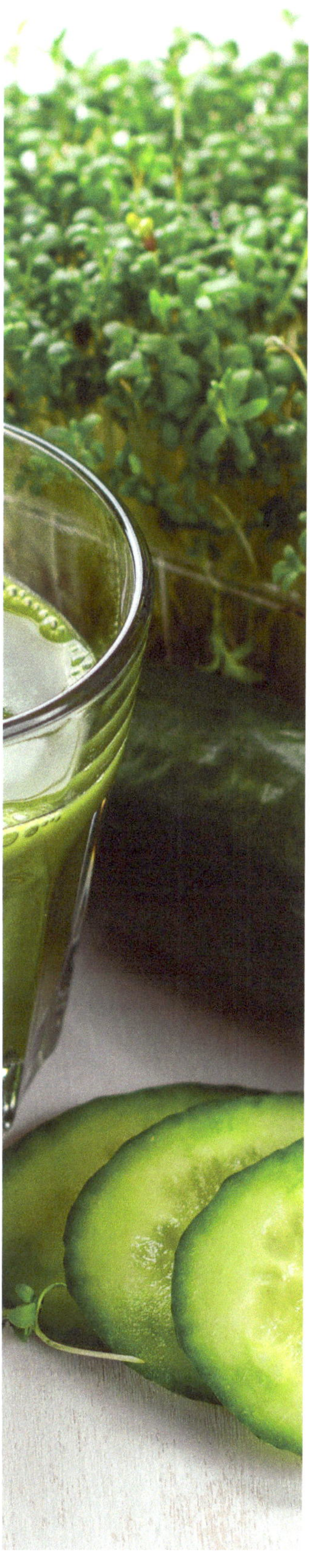

BANANA PEAR SMOOTHIE

Preparation time: 5 minutes
Serves: 2

Ingredients:
1 scoop protein powder
1 pear
1 apple (optional)
½ cup almond butter
2 bananas
8 oz dairy free yogurt
½ teaspoon of cinnamon

Directions: Mix together all ingredients in the blender. Pulse for 30 seconds on low speed, adjust to high and pulse until smooth. Serve immediately.

Nutrition Information (Per Serving):
Calorie: 265
Protein: 20.5g
Carbohydrate: 44.5g
Fat: 2.5g
Fiber: 6.5g
Sugar: 25g

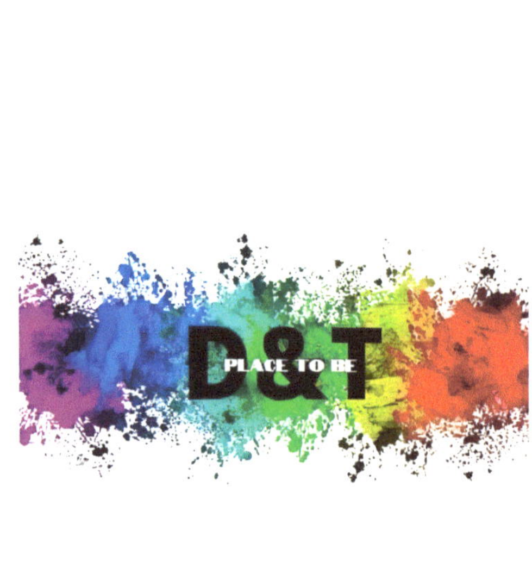

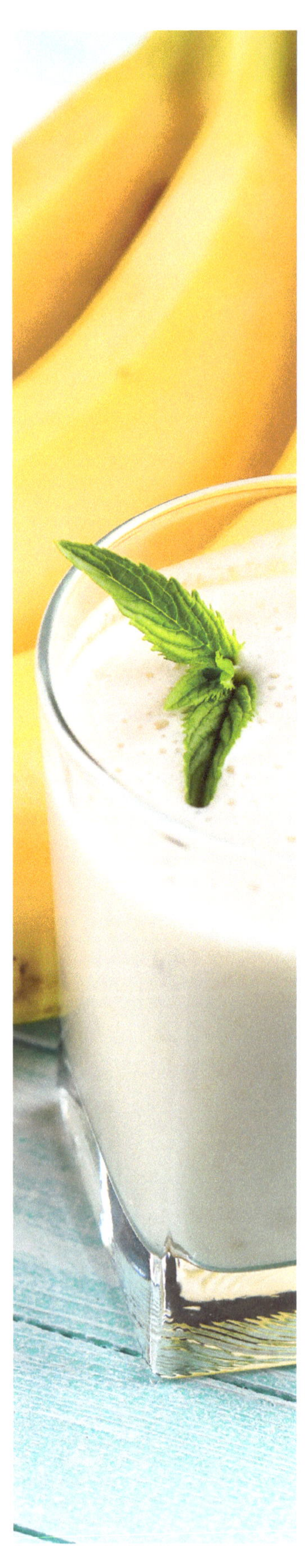

MIXED BERRY SMOOTHIE

Preparation time: 5 minutes
Serves: 2

Ingredients:
1 scoop pea protein powder
1 ½ cups frozen blueberry
½ cup frozen raspberries
½ cup frozen blackberries
2 tablespoon almond butter
1 ½ tablespoons raw honey
1 cup unsweetened almond Milk

Directions: Mix together all ingredients in the blender. Pulse for 30 seconds on low speed, adjust to high and pulse until smooth. Serve immediately.

Nutrition Information (Per Serving):
Calorie: 295.5
Protein: 14g
Carbohydrate: 40g
Fat: 11g
Fiber: 8g
Sugar: 23.5g

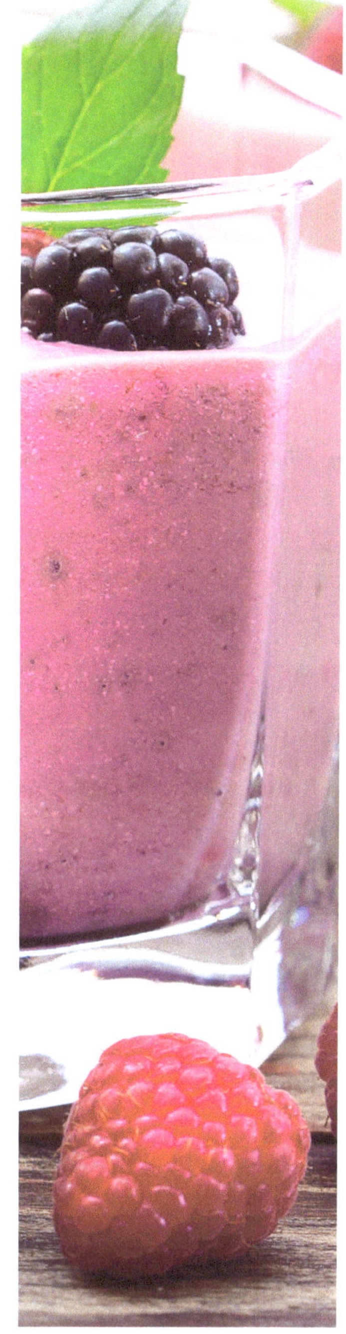

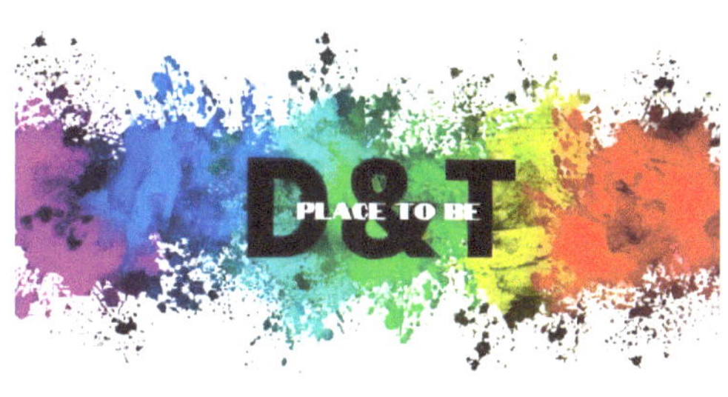

FRUITY MEAL SMOOTHIE

Preparation time: 5 minutes
Serves: 2

Ingredients:
1 banana, peeled
1 cup diced mango
4 large strawberries
1 cup dandelion greens
1 tablespoon flax seeds
1 scoop of protein powder
1 cup vanilla almond milk

Directions: Mix together all ingredients in the blender. Pulse for 30 seconds on low speed, adjust to high and pulse until smooth. Serve immediately.

Nutrition Information (Per Serving):
Calorie: 275.5
Protein: 4.7g
Carbohydrate: 44g
Fat: 44g
Fiber: 11.5g
Sugar: 28g

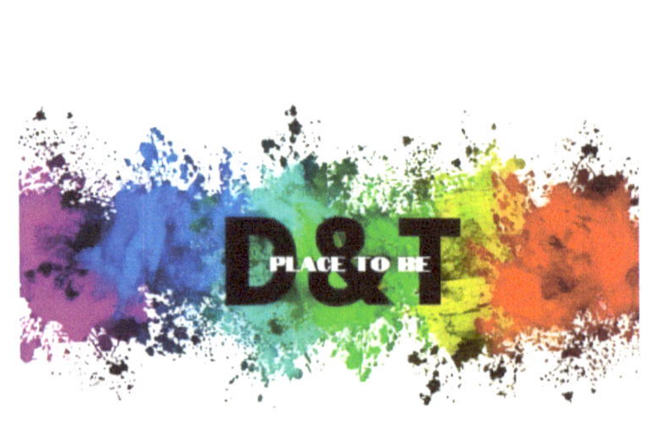

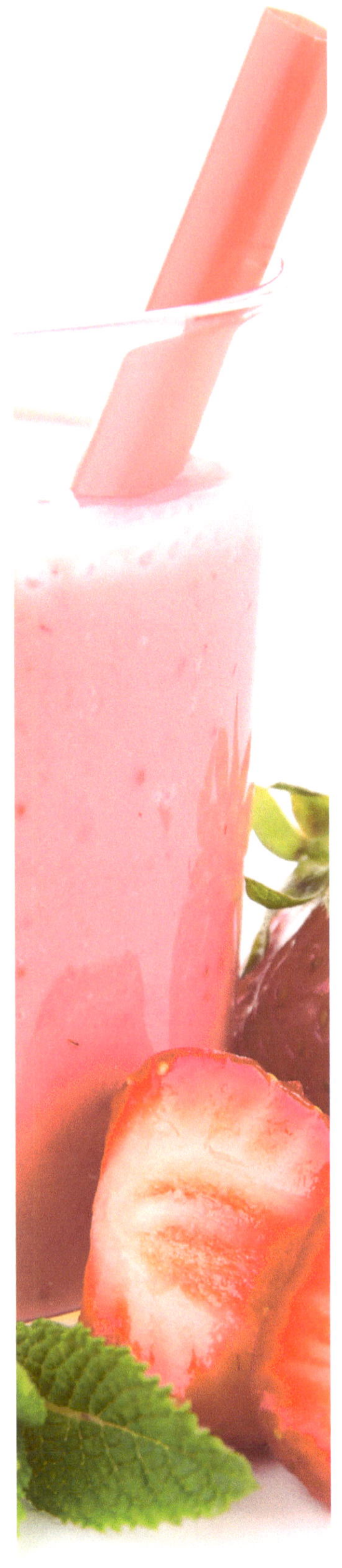

MIXED NUTS & SEEDS SMOOTHIE

Preparation time: 5 minutes
Serves: 2

Ingredients:
2 cups frozen strawberries
8 almonds
1 tablespoon chopped walnuts
1 tablespoon flax seed
1 tablespoon chia seed
1 scoop of protein powder
8 ounces of vanilla almond milk

Directions: Mix together all ingredients in the blender. Pulse for 30 seconds on low speed, adjust to high and pulse until smooth. Serve immediately.

Nutrition Information (Per Serving):
Calorie: 275.5
Protein: 17.5g
Carbohydrate: 23g
Fat: 13.5g
Fiber: 7.5g
Sugar: 12.5g

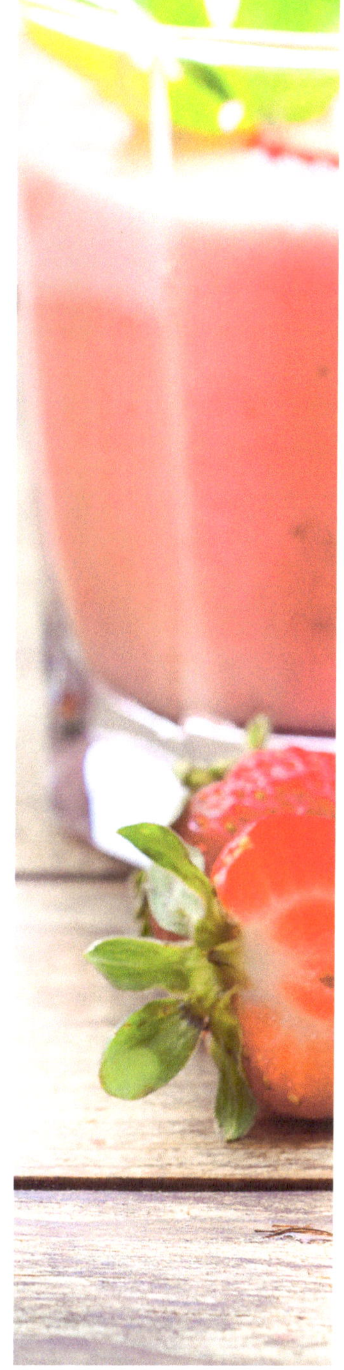

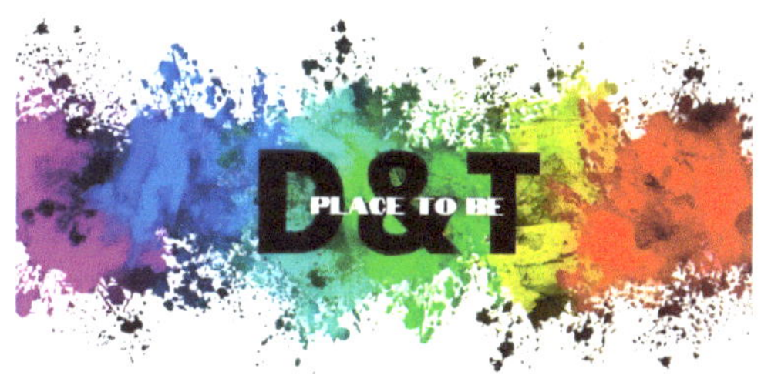

BANANA-STRAWBERRY SMOOTHIE

Preparation time: 5 minutes
Serves: 2

Ingredients:
1 cup vanilla almond milk
1 scoop protein powder
1 cup fresh spinach
1 banana
2 cups frozen strawberries
2 tablespoons old-fashioned rolled oats

Directions: Mix together all ingredients in the blender. Pulse for 30 seconds on low speed, adjust to high and pulse until smooth. Serve immediately.

Nutrition Information (Per Serving):
Calorie: 286.5
Protein: 17.5g
Carbohydrate: 47.5g
Fat: 4.4g
Fiber: 8g
Sugar: 26.5g

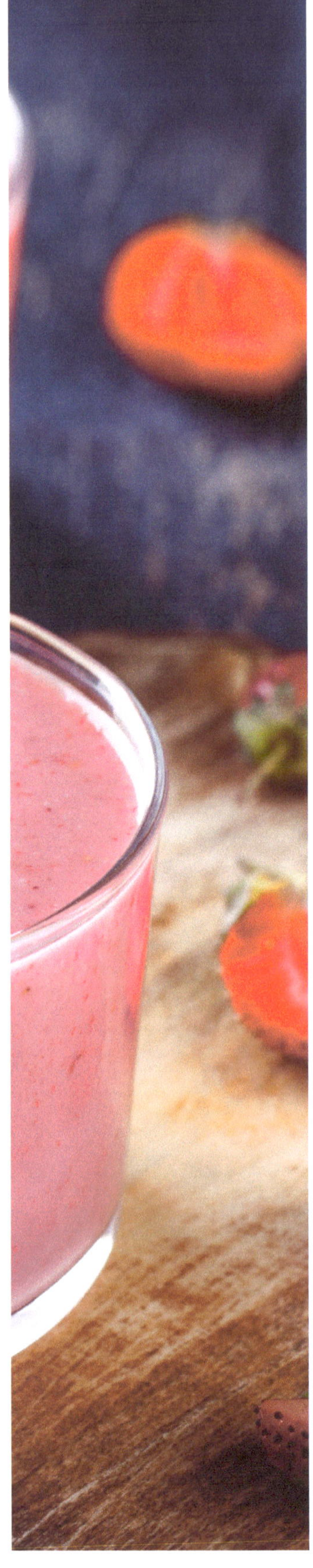

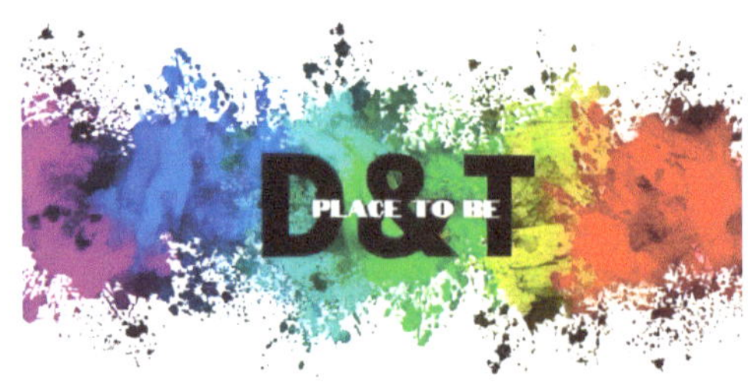

BLUEBERRY KALE SMOOTHIE

Preparation time: 5 minutes
Serves: 2

Ingredients:
4 ounces dairy free yogurt
1 scoop soy based protein powder
1 cup almond milk
20 pine nuts
1 cup loosely packed kale
2 cups frozen blueberries
1 tablespoon maple syrup

Directions: Mix together all ingredients in the blender. Pulse for 30 seconds on low speed, adjust to high and pulse until smooth. Serve immediately.

Nutrition Information (Per Serving):
Calorie: 292
Protein: 20.5g
Carbohydrate: 45.5g
Fat: 4.5g
Fiber: 6g
Sugar: 3.5g

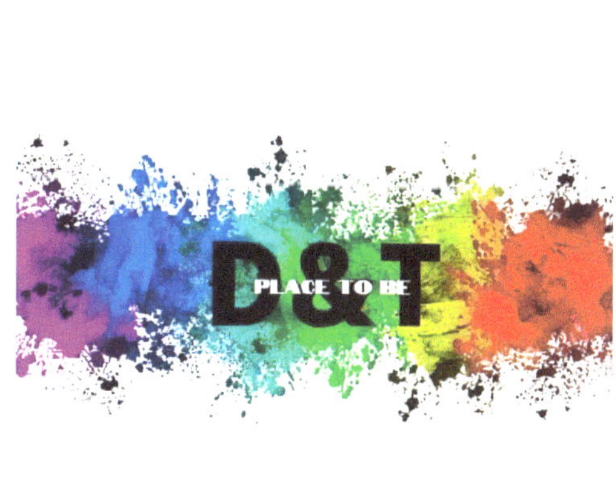

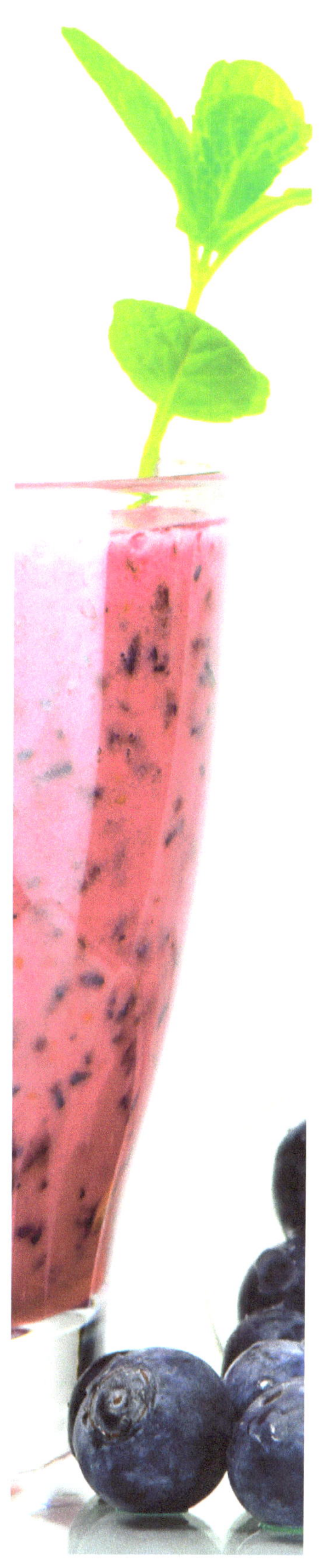

BANANA CARROT SMOOTHIE

Preparation time: 5 minutes
Serves: 2

Ingredients:
½ cup carrot juice
2 bananas
1 carrot
1 cup sweetened vanilla almond milk
1 scoop protein powder
½ teaspoon cinnamon

Directions: Mix together all ingredients in the blender. Pulse for 30 seconds on low speed, adjust to high and pulse until smooth. Serve immediately.

Nutrition Information (Per Serving):
Calorie: 275
Protein: 28g
Carbohydrate: 38.5g
Fat: 2.5g
Fiber: 5.5g
Sugar: 18g

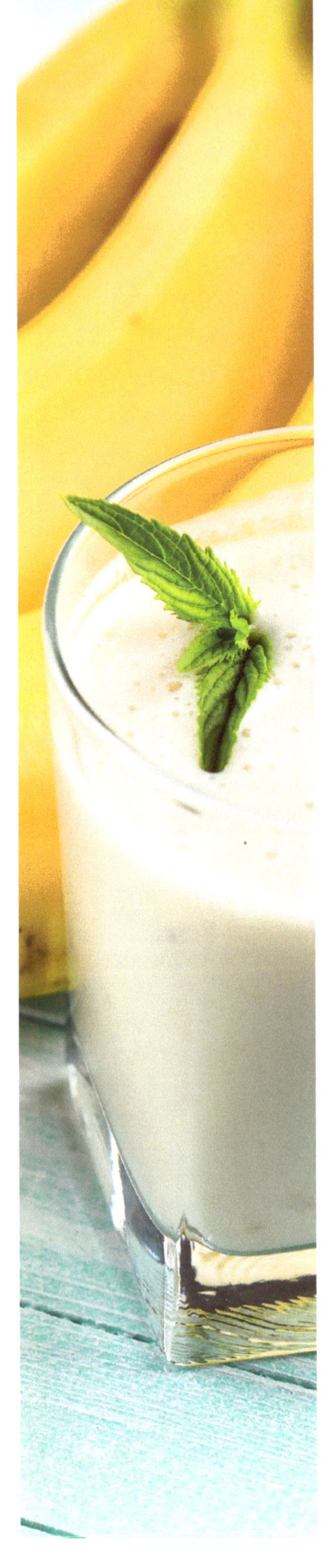

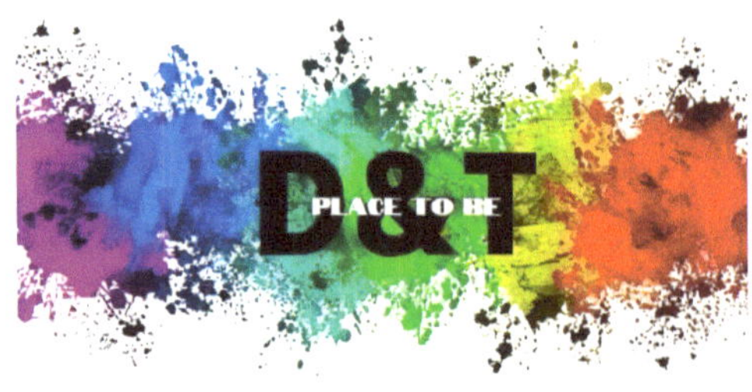

APPLE COCONUT SMOOTHIE

Preparation time: 5 minutes
Serves: 2

Ingredients:
6 ounces dairy free yogurt
½ cup shredded coconut meat
¼ cup almonds
½ teaspoon cinnamon
2 apples
1 scoop protein powder
1 tablespoon flax seeds

Directions: Mix together all ingredients in the blender. Pulse for 30 seconds on low speed, adjust to high and pulse until smooth. Serve immediately.

Nutrition Information (Per Serving):
Calorie: 298
Protein: 23.5g
Carbohydrate: 34.5g
Fat: 10g
Fiber: 8.5g
Sugar: 23g

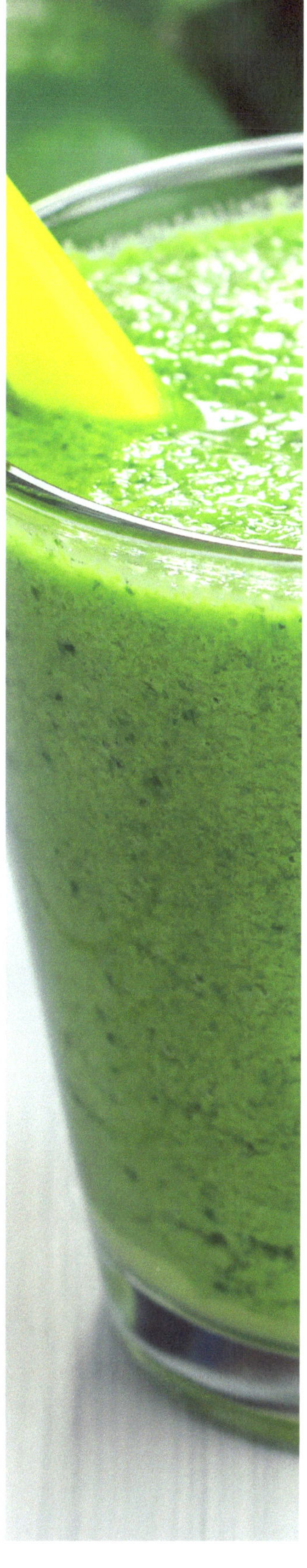

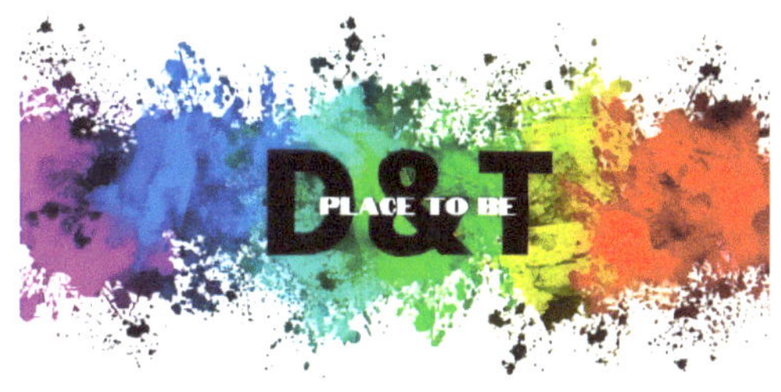

PUMPKIN PROTEIN SMOOTHIE

Preparation time: 5 minutes
Serves: 2

Ingredients:
1 cup dairy free yogurt
1 cup unsalted canned pumkin
1 ½ scoop protein powder
2 tablespoons cashew nuts
1 cup loosely packed kale
1 tablespoon raw honey
1 pinch of ground nutmeg

Directions: Mix together all ingredients in the blender. Pulse for 30 seconds on low speed, adjust to high and pulse until smooth. Serve immediately.

Nutrition Information (Per Serving):
Calorie: 280
Protein: 34.5g
Carbohydrate: 21.5g
Fat: 7.5g
Fiber: 5.5g
Sugar: 9g

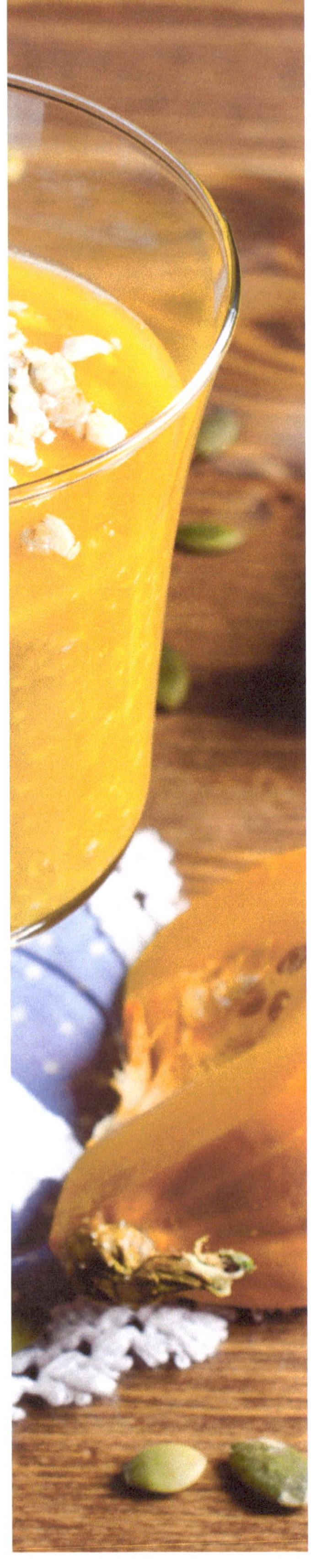

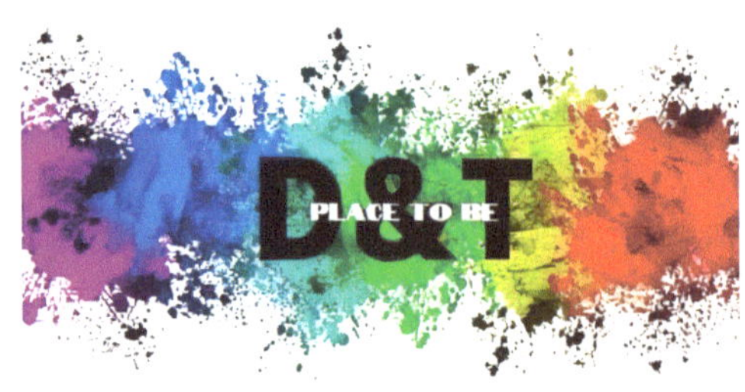

GRAPE SPINACH SMOOTHIE

Preparation time: 5 minutes
Serves: 2

Ingredients:
2 cups seedless frozen green grapes
2 cups of spinach
½ cup coconut water
1 cup dairy free yogurt
2 tablespoons chia seeds
1 tablespoon of raw honey

Directions: Mix together all ingredients in the blender. Pulse for 30 seconds on low speed, adjust to high and pulse until smooth. Serve immediately.

Nutrition Information (Per Serving):
Calorie: 290
Protein: 16.5g
Carbohydrate: 45.5g
Fat: 5.5g
Fiber: 7.5g
Sugar: 27.5g

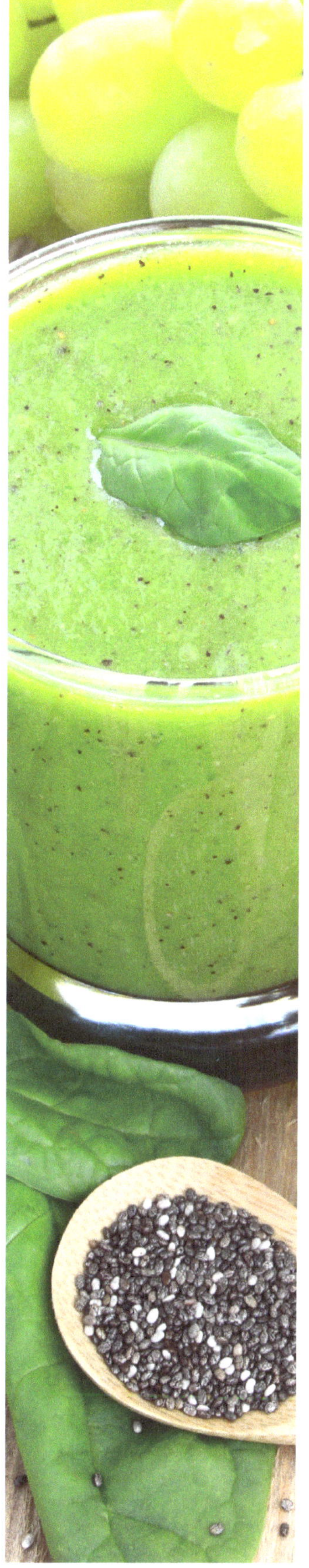

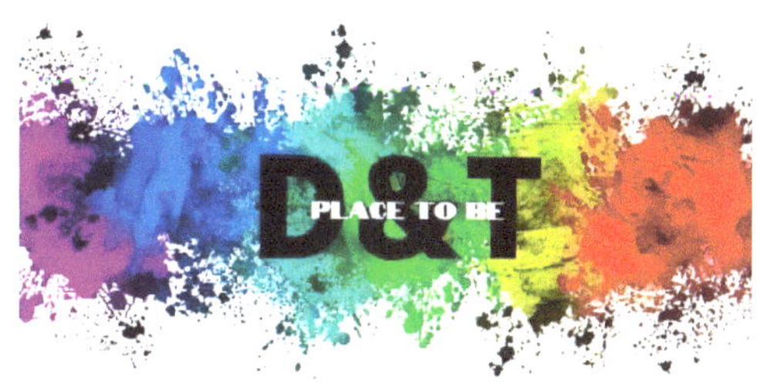